CONSUMING WITH A CONSCIENCE

&

RAISING CONSCIOUS KIDS

A PLANET-BASED FAMILY FRIENDLY GUIDE

JOANNA WALKER

Consuming with a Conscience and Raising Conscious Kids

ISBN: 978-0-578-23156-3

Interior Formatting/Design by Amit Dey | amitdey2528@gmail.com

TABLE OF CONTENTS

The beginning: The inspiration behind "Consuming with a Conscience and raising conscious Kids." A Plant Based book.

Chapter 1

INTRODUCTION

Firstly, I would like to Thank you the reader for purchasing my book. I pray that it helps you along your Plant based Journey. Whether it's to get new ideas for you or your child that's already on a plant-based diet or if it's because you want to raise your newborns on a plant based diet. The recipes in this book is for adults too, but kid friendly, as I know kids can sometimes be fussy eaters. Choosing a Plant-Based diet for your child is one of the best things you could do for them, and I promise they will Thank you for it.

It all starts with simple things such as food, I was taught that "food could be your medicine or it could be your poison". What you put in your body is so important, and we need to teach our children that from the very beginning.

Prevention is always better than cure, so taking the initiative to learn the necessary information, to better support your children, is great.

So, well doe Mommy and Daddy!

Over years of studying, I have learned that diets, over eating and meat consumption are all things that have been spoken about in the bible. There's been many scriptures that warn us about being aware of what we eat. This brings me to the topic of how eating certain foods can also influence you spiritually.

Helping your children grow into conscious human beings, is so beneficial. Especially in the world we live in today.

MY STORY

My Plant-based Journey began when I had my first child in 2013. Ever since I was young, I was always put off from the idea of eating animals. I never liked seeing raw meat, and often was put off if I saw some-thing that I didn't like. This narrowed me down to only consuming Fish and chicken.

September 2013, I came across a documentary that answered a lot of questions for me regarding food. I learned a lot about the behind scenes of the food practically the "meat" industry.

This then sparked my first steps in to transitioning to a vegan diet.

My husband also embarked on this Journey with me, but it only lasted for about 3-4 months. We didn't know much about plant-based diet and often ran out of recipe ideas, places to find these ingredients that wasn't out of the way. Not forgetting to mention not having food options, when we went out to eat, attended events, birthdays and family get togethers.

This lead us back to consuming fish and chicken, however we completely cut out dairy and eggs.

In the beginning of 2015, I was pregnant with my second child. During this year I had what some may call a "Spiritual Awakening". I was doing a lot soul searching trying to figure out what my actual purpose was. It all became clear when I got a message from my mother, saying she had a message for me after praying one day. This was confirmation that natural health was the path for me.

After having my daughter, I remember having questions, lots of questions regarding my own health. Whenever I ate, I would feel uncomfortable, it was like my stomach was always irritated. This is a feeling I had for years, however I learned to ignore. I have mentioned this issue to Dr's but it was always brushed off.

When my daughter was about 2-3 months old, she started to suffer from constipation. As a mother, it was heartbreaking to see her go through that. I had to take a step back and analyze the situation. I was breast-feeding, so this only meant that I wasn't doing something right.

After research, I completely changed my diet to a plant-based diet, I also made sure all my ingredients were alkaline and organic.

Incorporating lots of more leafy greens.

Not only did the constipation stop, but my stomach irritation did too.

Ever since then, I have been rising my children on a plant-based diet and hope that one day soon my husband will also join our journey.

After my experience I decided to study natural health and holistic nutrition. This is what lead me to where I am today.

I am writing this to help guide anyone that gets stuck along the way. In 2013, when me and my husband tried a plant-based diet for the first time, we didn't have much quick resources to refer to. Who knows, maybe if we did have a compact guide with recipes, tips and knowledge, we would have all stayed on that path from then.

I hope this book is healthful to you and your family.

Wishing you Peace, Love and Happiness.

Lots of Love,
Joanna Walker

What is Plant- Based/ Vegan? A plant-based diet consists of fruits, vegetables, whole grains and legumes. A Vegan diet consist of the same except, they are a little more strict. They will not consume or use any animal products what so ever. This also includes the use of honey, products tested on animals, clothing and shoes.

Chapter 2

MY REASON'S TO BE PLANT-BASED OR VEGAN.

Health - "A good diet is the most basic human need. without enough nourishing food, we would die" (Food and Nutrition). Studies have proven that living on a plant-based diet is the best route for optimal health. People who eat a plant based nutritious Whole Foods, live a longer life span, rarely ever get sick, and over all are happier and healthier. Humans are naturally Herbivores; we were never designed to eat meat. Our anatomy was never made to consume animal flesh, our teeth, our digestive tracts, stomachs PH, are different to animals who consume meat. I always used the scenario of a premium car versus a standard car. If you put premium gas into a standard car, it will still run. However, that does not mean you are not doing damage on the inside, eventually that car will break down from the simply not putting in the correct fuel. This is where disease come in to play. Studies prove that eating a meat free diet reduces the risk of disease. The mistake most people make when transitioning in to a plant- based diet is eating a vegan version on of the Standard American Diet.

Therefore, you may find some vegans that are overweight, nutrient deficient, or get sick often. Therefore, it is important to choose whole plant-based foods and stay away from processed Junk.

Animals - Animals are friends not food. All animals including fish (yes, A fish is an animal) are living, breathing and Thinking creations of God. All animals are equal, No different from your pet dog or cat. Everyday billions of innocent animals such as cows, pigs and chickens are tortured, abused and killed. These animals feel emotions just as we do. Most of these animals are crowded into muddy feces filled sheds, never being able to see natural sunlight, or breath fresh air. Chicken's never gotten to spread their wings as they are in crowded small spaces. Cows are taken away from their babies straight after birth and hooked up to milking machines. The baby calves don't even have a chance to feed from their own mother. The calves are then sold to the veal industry. After 5- 6 years of what should be a 20 plus year life span, the mother cow is worn out from the excessive milk pumping and birth after births. They are then sent to slaughter. Studies have proven that even fish feel pain and fear. It has been said that the rapid pressure change causes their swim bladders to rapture and causes their eyes to pop out. Most Fish die from slow suffocation or from being cut up alive.

More than 50% of fish today is farm raised, where they live in filthy conditions and suffer from parasitic infections and many diseases.

Even Exotic rainforest Animals suffer from the consumption of animal flesh. Many of these beautiful animals have become extinct due to deforestation.

Spiritual- When disease strikes, you often hear people blame God. My Question is why? Regardless of your religious beliefs, all religions have rules about eating.

If you go back to Genesis, you will learn that the first diet God gave us was a plant-based diet. Since the very beginning our bodies have not evolved to eat otherwise. Even studies of biology show that humans are, by anatomy and physiology frugivores, and remain species of vegetarians. I personally came across a few passages in the bible, where it speaks about, us needing to be aware of the type of food we eat, because the type of food we ingest may be tainted with dangerous bacteria and toxins. (Colossians 2:8) when eating animal flesh, you are allowing your body to be invaded by unwanted invaders. (Parasites) These entities can control your mood, thoughts and cravings. They survive by using you or another living thing as a host. (2 Corinthians 7:1) "Let us cleanse ourselves from all filthiness that contaminated and defiles the flesh and spirit, perfecting holiness in God's fear". Keeping your body physically clean on the inside and out, symbolizes high a level of spirituality before the eyes of God. (Leviticus 11:41-47) There was certain laws that considered one as unclean after eating certain birds, fish and animals. Many people I've spoken to who have engaged in some sort of spiritual contact, have all mention one thing in common. The message they have received was to eliminate meat and consume Just fruit and vegetables. (Daniel 1:11-21) A vegetarian diet is superior to a flesh-eating diet".

We need be aware that the foods we eat can defile our flesh and pollute our blood.

The Bible states animals have souls. The exact Hebrew word used in reference to animals throughout the Bible is "nephesh chayah," or "living soul." This is how the phrase has been translated in (Genesis 2:7) and in many other places in the Old Testament. Thus, (Genesis 1:30) should more accurately read: "And to every beast of the earth, and to every fowl of the air, and to everything that creepeth upon the earth, wherein there is a living soul, I have given every green herb for meat."

God breathed the "breath of life" into man and caused him to become a living soul. (Genesis 2:7) Animals have the same "breath of life" as do humans. (Genesis 7:15, 22) (Numbers 16:22) refers to the Lord as "the God of spirits of all flesh." In (Numbers 31:28), God commands Moses to divide up among the people the cattle, sheep, asses and human prisoners captured in battle and to give to the Lord "one soul of five hundred" of both humans and animals alike. {Psalm 104} says God provides for animals and their ensoulment.

So, you must ask yourself, If God intended for us to consume animal flesh, 3 or more times a day, as some people do.

Why doesn't our body process it? Why do we generate diseases in our bodies? Why does it create the environment for parasites to thrive? Then ask yourself, why does eating Fruits, Vegetables and herbs, heal, electrify, nourish, build and ground us?

(Genesis 1:29) "God said, I give you every seed-Bearing plant on the face of the earth and every tree has fruit with seed in, this shall be yours for food".

Environment- Studies show that we have entered our 6th mass extinction of species with an average of 50% of land degradation in the past 50 years. Millions of acres of rainforest burned every year just to make pasture for grazing animals. More than 50% of water supply goes towards raising animals for food, and in reverse animal waste pollutes more water sources than any other industry. We have caused devastation to our oceans as we pump insane amounts of plastic destroying our ocean and sea life, we pump extreme amounts of green House gases into the atmosphere, leading to global warming, also warming our oceans leading to coral reef dying and Storms after storms. All this destruction due to the mass consumption of animals and animal products. There must come a point where the life of animals is worth more than your taste. The World must Acknowledge that and choose compassion.

(Revolution 11:18) God will bring to ruin those who ruining the earth.

(Isaiah 24:5-6) The land has been polluted under its inhabitants, and those inhabiting it are held guilty.

Chapter 3

ESSENTIAL VITAMINS

VITAMIN B-12

Vitamin B-12 is important to maintain healthy nerve cells. It supports energy, protects the heart, protects brain health, prevents nerve damage and even improves mood.

Most people think that you can only get Vitamin B-12 from animal products. The truth is B-12 is synthesized by bacteria and is found in areas of bacteria growth, such as soil and dirt. When animals eat from the ground, it also consumes the B-12. When the animal is consumed by humans the B-12 from the animal flesh or milk, is also ingested. If a vegan had a few unwashed vegetables, B-12 will also be consumed with those veggies. However, Vegetables and fruit always need to be washed, to keep clear from contaminants and parasites.

Vitamin B12 Dosages				
Age	US RDA (µg)	2 Doses per Day (µg)	Daily Dose (µg)	2 Doses per Week (µg)
0 - 5 months	0.4	n/a	n/a	n/a
6 - 11 months	0.4	0.4 - 1	5 - 20	200
1 - 3 yrs	0.9	0.8 - 1.5	10 - 40	375
4 - 8 yrs	1.2	1 - 2	13 - 50	500
9 - 13 yrs	1.8	1.5 - 2.5	20 - 75	750
14 - 64 yrs	2.4	2 - 3.5	25 - 100	1000
65+ yrs.	2.6	-	500 - 1000	-
Pregnancy	2.6	2.5 - 4	25 - 100	1000
Lactation	2.8	2.5 - 4	30 - 100	1000

µg = mcg = microgram = 1/1,000 of a milligram (mg)

n/a - Not applicable. Infants should be receiving breast milk or commercial
formula which contains the necessary amounts of vitamin B12.

There is a large difference between amounts taken twice daily and once daily because beyond 3 µg (for adults), absorption drops significantly.

Amounts much larger than these are considered safe, but it's probably best not to take more than twice the recommended amounts.

AThese recommendations are for cyanocobalamin only. There is not enough research on other forms of vitamin B12 to recommend specific dosages from supplements. For more information, see Alternatives to Cyanocobalamin: Methylcobalamin & Dibencozide.

Many Plant based milks are Vitamin B-12 fortified, so be sure to check all your plant-based labels to see, if it already contains B-12.

Otherwise you can always supplement with brands Like Veg Life vegan kid's multivitamins, Global Healing or The Honest co, just to name a few.

I have provided a recommended dosage chart above. Please speak to your child's physician if you have any questions or concerns about the right dosage.

OMEGA 3

Omega 3's help reduce Inflammation. Inflammation is the root cause of many health problems, so getting the right nutrient balance is important. Omega-3 fats are also abundant in brain cells, nerve synapses, visual receptors, adrenal glands making it vital to a child's normal growth and development. Omega-3 fats are critical to keeping a child's brain and body in biochemical balance and providing children with the building blocks for a strong immune system.

There are many great Vegan sources of Omega 3's, so you don't have to eat fish or take fish oil to get them. You can make sure your child is getting those omegas 3's in their diets by, simply adding sources such as, flaxseeds to their porridge or smoothies.

Other Vegan friendly sources are:

Avocados, Chia seeds, Hemp seeds, Walnuts, Brussel sprouts, flaxseed oil, hempseed oil and chia seed oil.

The U.S. Food and Drug Administration established daily values, or DVs, for total fat and saturated fat but has not yet established daily values for polyunsaturated fats like omega-3. The Food and Nutrition Board of the Institute of Medicine, National Academy of Sciences established dietary reference intake or DRI for ALA for individuals based on age and sex. The ALA DRIs range from 500 mg for infants up to 1,600 mg per day for males aged 14 to 18. The U.S. Department of Agriculture, Food and Nutrition Information Center website provides an interactive tool to determine DRIs for dietary planning. The tool determines the DRI for the nutrients listed, including ALA, based on the personal information provided. Dr. Sears, in "The NDD Book," recommends different dosages for different ages. For infants, the recommended dose is at least 300 mg per day. For children ages 2 to 3, at least 400 mg per day is recommended. For children over 4, the recommended dose is at least 600 mg per day. Some health care providers recommend a higher therapeutic dose of up to 1,000 mg a day for children with autism, ADD, ADHD or learning disabilities.

VITAMIN C

Vitamin C is known to help support and boost the immune system, it also helps with the growth, development and repair of all body tissues. Vitamin C is necessary and involved in many body functions, including formation of collagen, absorption of iron, the immune system, wound healing, and the maintenance of cartilage, bones, and teeth.

Great Vegan friendly sources of Vitamin C are:

Kiwi fruit, Oranges, Cherries, Raspberries, Lemon, Lime, Pineapple, papayas, guava, strawberries, mango Kale, Spinach and bell peppers.

IRON

Iron is important for the blood, it's a component of hemoglobin. Hemoglobin is the substance in the red blood cells responsible for, carrying oxygen, from your lungs throughout your body. Iron is what helps your body make enough healthy oxygen carrying red blood cells.

Great Vegan friendly sources for iron are:

Spinach, lentils, Baked Potato, Beans, Quinoa and Broccoli.

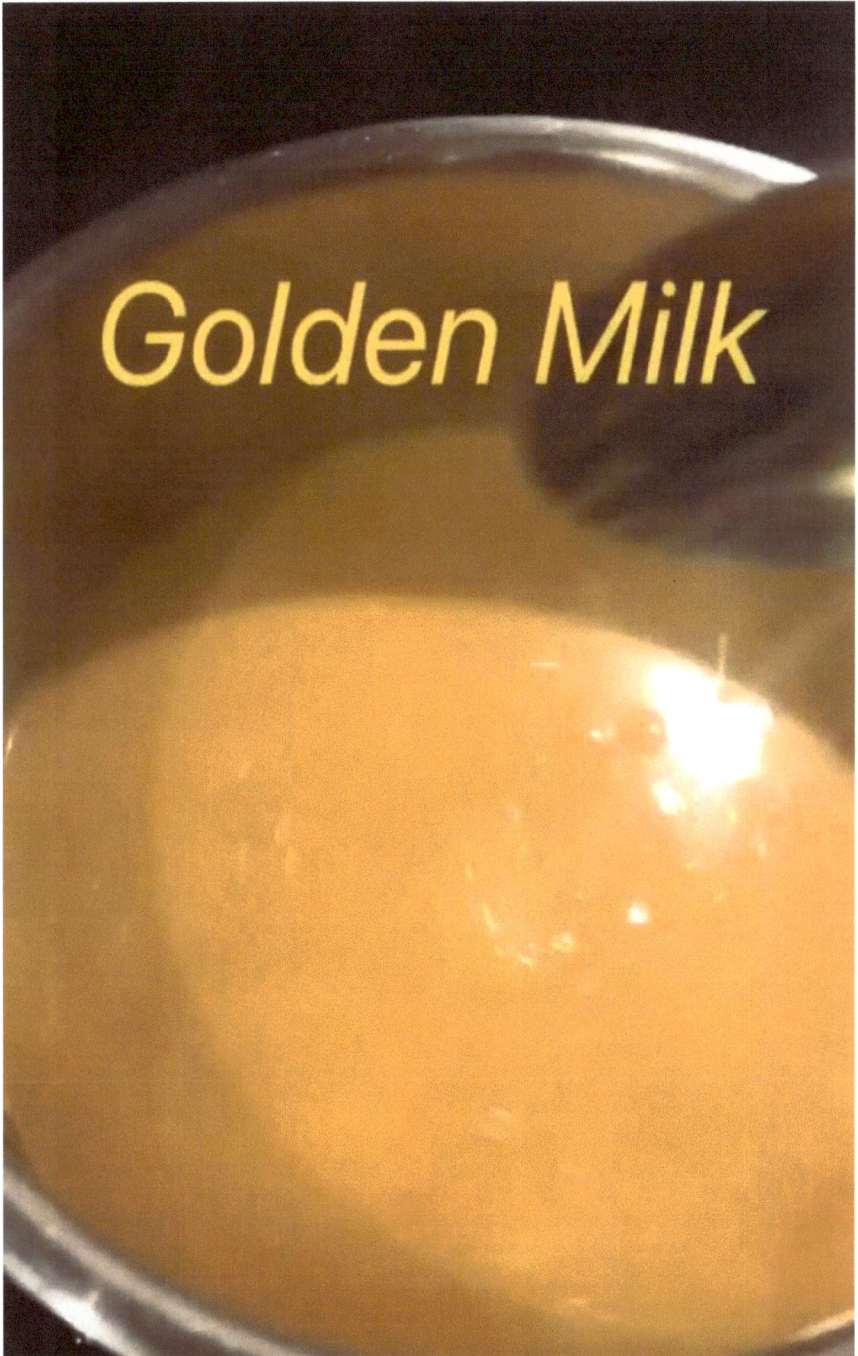

Golden Milk

Chapter 4

IMMUNE BOOSTING TIPS

The white blood cells are the prime cells of the immune system. They defend the body by fighting against infectious diseases and foreign invaders. To support the white blood cells, consuming the right supporting foods and herbs are essential. I choose not to vaccinate, so building and maintaining a healthy immune system is very important to me.

MY TOP TIPS FOR A HEALTHY IMMUNE SYSTEM.

1. **Lemon, ginger, Turmeric Shot**

   - 1 Lemon
   - 1 tsp agave

- 1 ½ tsp ground ginger
- 1½ tsp Turmeric
- 100 ml spring water

2. **Elderberry glycerite drops** (Herb Pharm kid's) Put a drop in 2oz juice, water or smoothie 2-4 times a day.

3. **Golden Milk-** The perfect anti-inflammatory drink before bed.

   - 200ml organic Coconut Milk
   - 1 tbsp Turmeric
   - 1 tsp ginger
   - 1 tsp nutmeg
   - ½ tsp cinnamon
   - 1 tbsp Agave

Diffusers and Pink Himalayan Lamps are also great tools for night time immune boosting.

If you choose to use a diffuser, my favorite immune boosting essential oils are:

- Lemon oil
- Clove oil
- Eucalyptus oil

- Rosemary oil
- Lavender oil
- Frankincense oil

Pink Himalayan lamps have many great benefits, this mineral miracle is made from the purist salt crystals. These are some of the reason's you should have a pink Himalayan salt lamp in your home:

- Immune system enhancement
- Neutralizes electromagnetic radiation
- Eases coughing
- Reduces allergy and asthma symptoms
- Cleanses and deodorizes the air
- improves sleep
- Improves mood and concentration
- Environmentally friendly light source

PROBIOTICS

Probiotics are very beneficial for your little one's immune system. It has been said that most of the immune system is in the gut. So good microbe balance is essential for keeping the Immune strong and ready to fight off any colds or illnesses.

Providing your kid's with nutrient-dense whole foods such as vegetables, fruits, nuts, and ancient grains is a great way to help maintain healthy levels of good bacteria in the gut. Include prebiotic-rich foods into the diet on daily basis helps maintain a healthily balanced gut microbiome Foods such as bananas, apples, artichokes, asparagus, and onions contain special fibers called prebiotics that help feed the good bacteria in the gut.

Research has shown that giving children probiotics, both through food and supplements can improve overall health. A few other benefits for your child besides healthy immune may include:

- Improved Mood and behavior
- Healthy Bowel Movement
- Good Brain Function
- Healthy Weight
- Healthy metabolism

Giving a probiotic supplement regularly helps boost levels of good bacteria and supports healthy brain and body function. It is important to use quality products that are formulated to survive harsh stomach acid in order to make it to the intestines where they belong. Stay away from probiotic products containing sugar or artificial ingredients such as dyes or flavorings, as these ingredients work to cancel out the benefits of taking probiotic supplements. The Brand that I found most useful is from Garden of Life Dr's formulated, Organic Kid's probiotics. They have a variety of natural flavor's, which taste great the kids love them as they are chewable. This brand has no added sugar, artificial flavors, sweeteners, colors or preservatives.

BLACK SEED OIL

Black seed oil is like nature's cough syrup. It soothes as it strengthens. I feel like moment you take a spoonful is the moment you can officially say goodbye to anything attacking your immune system. It's one of the best natural ways to build a strong immune system. This oil is primarily effective in fighting various forms of bacterial infection. Black cumin seed oil boosts your body's natural killer cells. These cells are critical to your well-being. Natural killer cells are a type of white blood cell that seek out and destroy viruses. They also respond to tumor formation. Amazingly, black cumin seed oil has been proven to wipe out harmful bacteria where antibiotic medications cannot. As a natural anti-bacterial agent, it can fight against many bacteria that are either immune or resistant to conventional pharmaceutical interventions. Over time

It has become popular with the discovery of various health benefits and immune system perks that can be achieved with Just a small dose. Me and My kids have our daily dose before bed, it's not the best tasting, so I let the kids have some water or a sip of fresh Juice to chase it down. I found that the more consistent we are, the more their taste buds adjust, to the point they do not need any chasers.

Black Seed Oil has amazing health benefits which includes:

- Improving immune function
- Balancing cholesterol
- Fighting infections
- Fighting harmful pathogens
- Reducing inflammation
- Improving cognitive performance
- Supporting liver health
- Improving skin health,
- Supporting eye health
- Supporting hair growth
- Removes Mucus

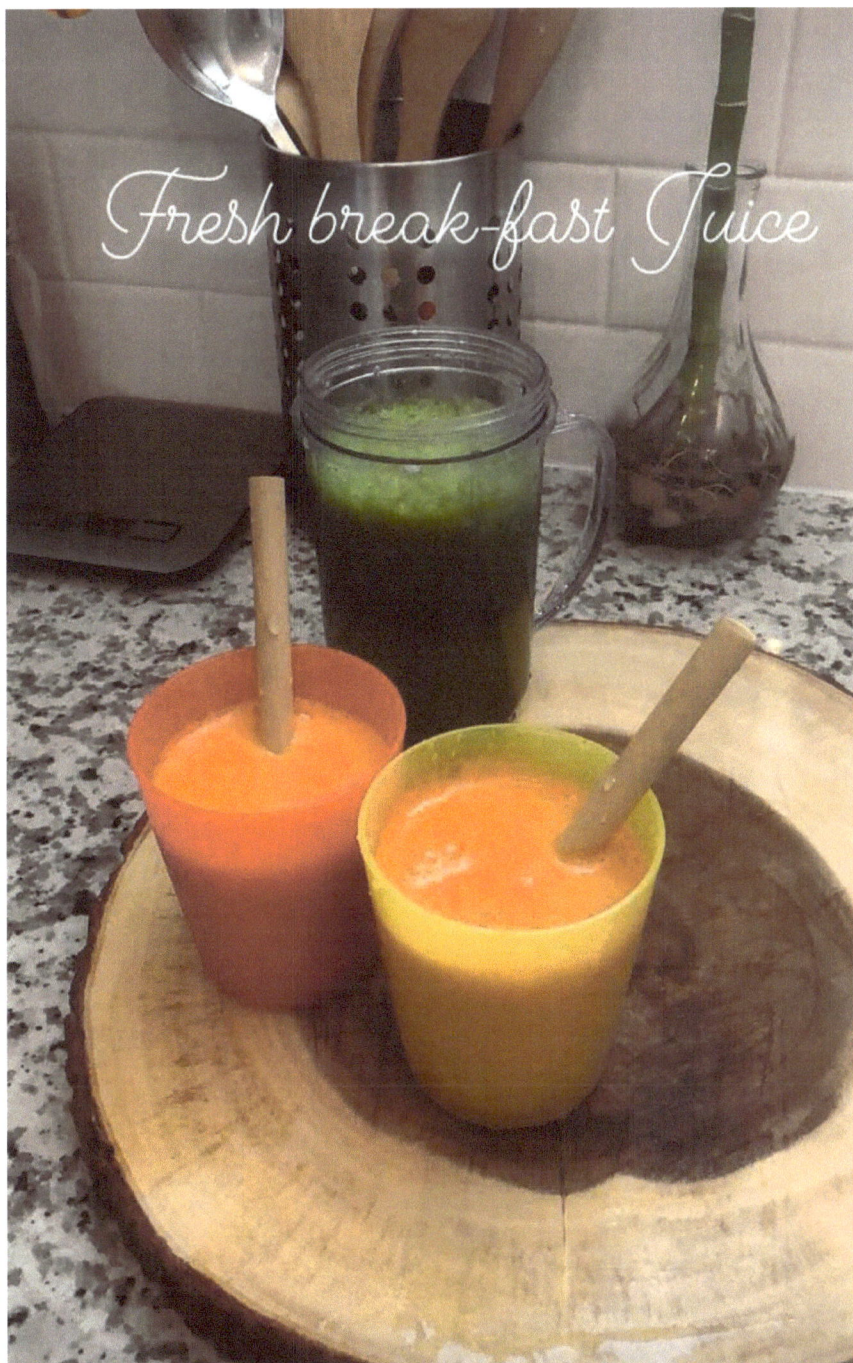

Fresh break-fast Juice

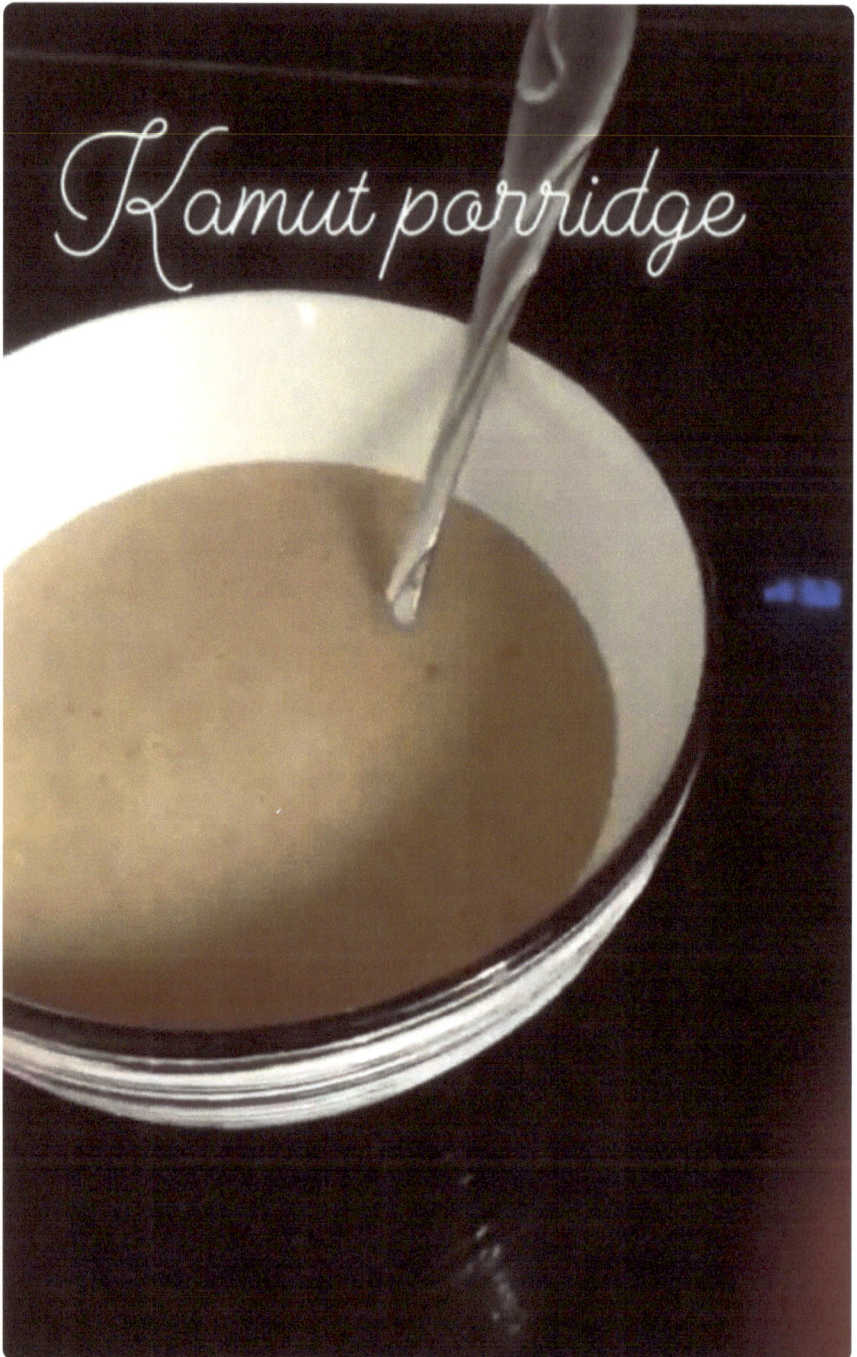

Kamut porridge

Chapter 5

JUICING

Juicing is a great way to ensure your kids are getting enough of their vitamins and minerals from raw vegetables and fresh fruit.

I also find that it's a great way to sneak in any vegetables that they may not like or eat whole on its own.

It's best to start the day with a cup or glass of water or fresh Juice. Ideally, the first thing you consume in the morning should be water, fruit or leafy greens.

The reason for this leafy vegetables, fruit and herbs require the least amount of digestive energy. These foods have their own digestive enzymes, which prevents any digestive stress on the body. It also gives your body more energy to kick start your day, as all the immune boosting nutrients is absorbed faster.

I was so lucky to be gifted with an awesome juicer for my Birthday. It's an essential item, especially in a vegan kitchen.

HERE IS MY TOP 4 JUICE BLENDS.

Note: Remove all large seeds before Juicing. I normally peel the skin off some fruits such mango, oranges and melons.

1. Mango, Papaya, Apple and Orange
2. Celery, Kale, apple and cucumber and Lime
3. Red grapes and Concord Grapes
4. Watermelon

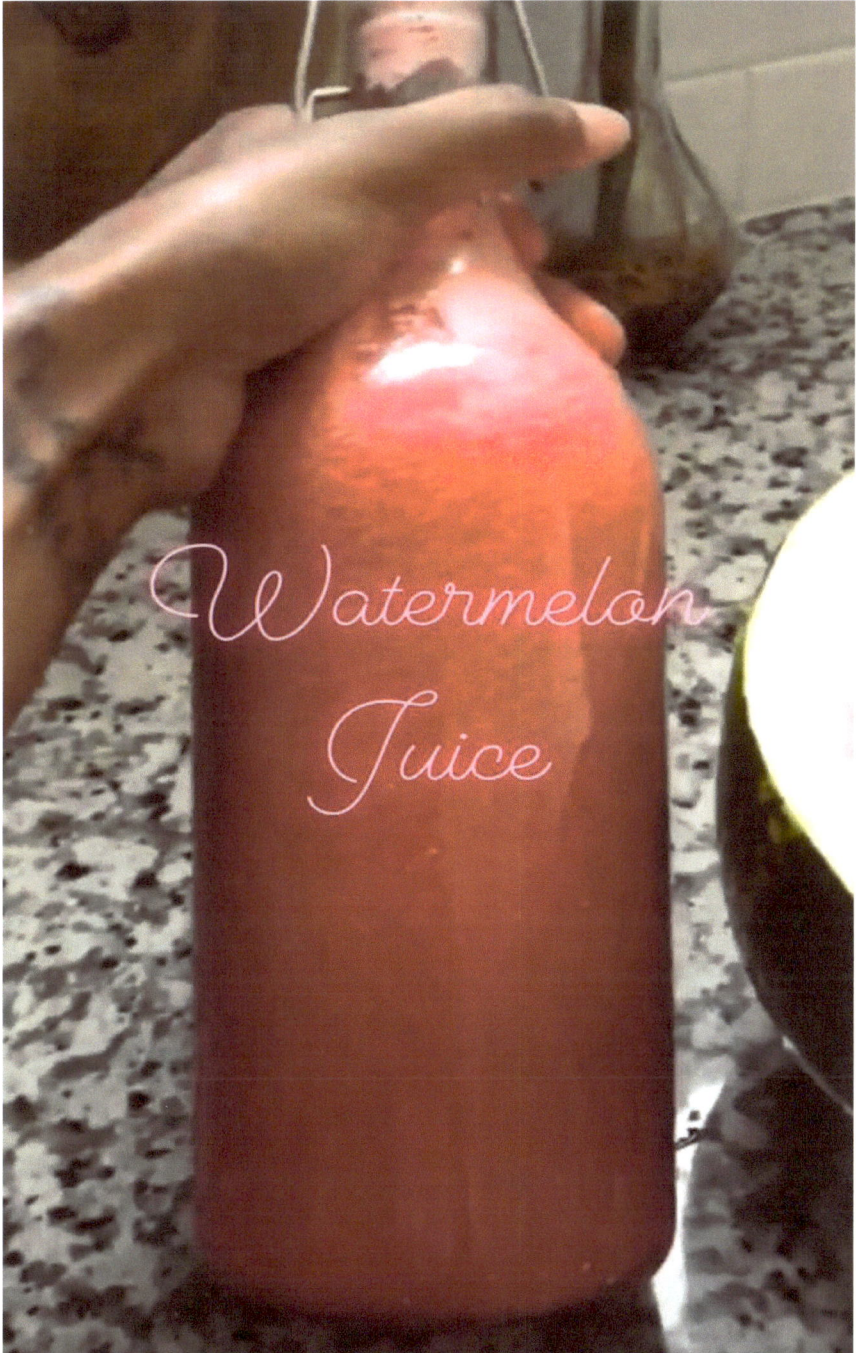

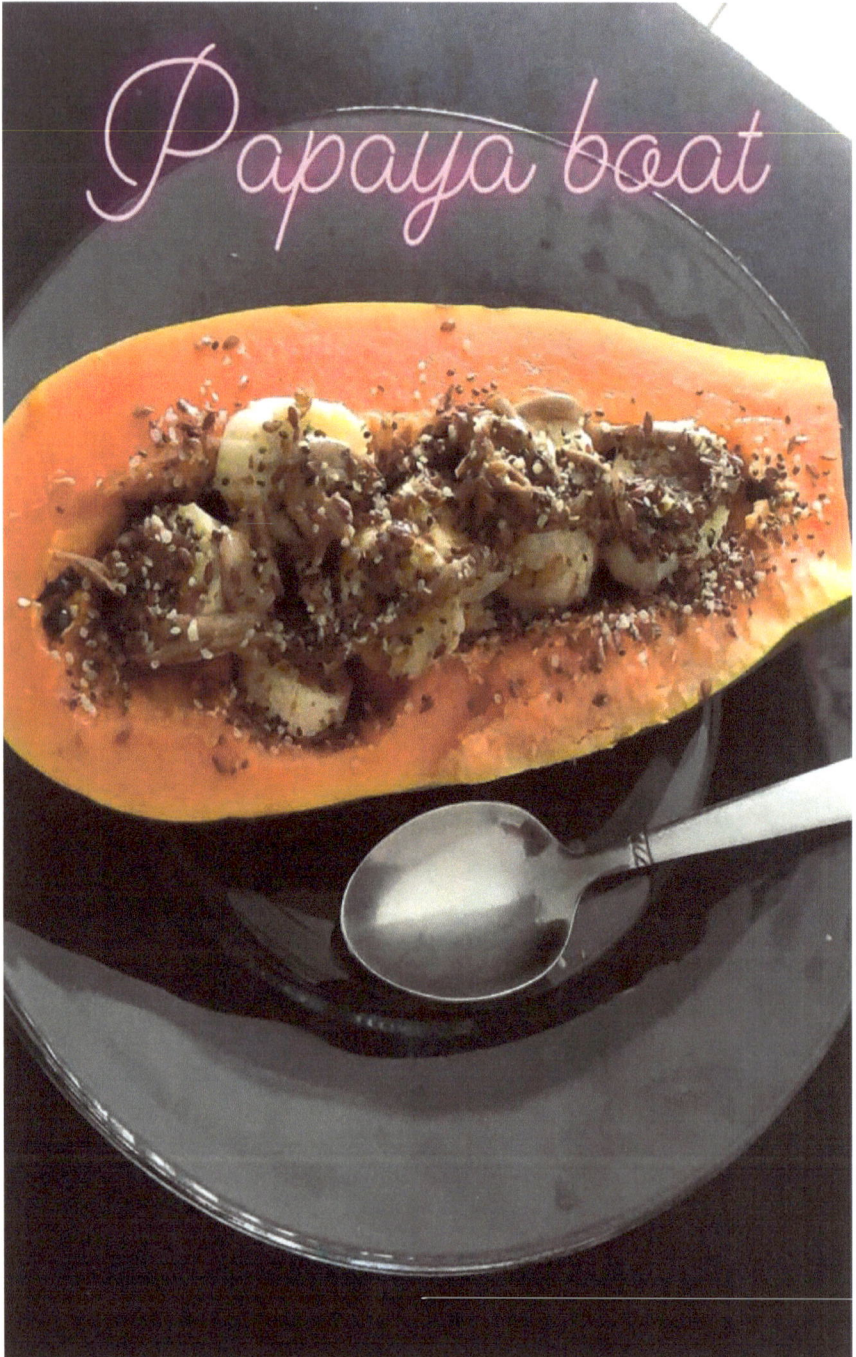

Papaya boat

Chapter 6

7 DAYS OF PLANT-BASED BREAKFAST

B reakfast is said to be the most important meal of the day. What you fuel your body with to kick start your day is important.

The first thing you consume in the morning should in fact be water, fresh fruit, or fresh fruit and green leafy vegetable Juice. The reason for this is because whilst you are asleep your body is taking a break from consuming anything. This is also considering fasting. When you initially break a fast, you break it with either water of fruit. A deeper explanation of this, is in my "Juicing" chapter.

Once you and your kids have had your Juice, water or fresh fruit. I have provided 7 breakfast/ Brunch Ideas below. Some of which you can essentially have as your first meal or drink of the day.

1. Avocado Spelt Flat Bread

Ingredients:

- Spelt Flour
- Mixed Herbs
- Pink Himalayan Sea Salt
- Spring Water
- ½ lime
- 1 large Avocado
- Black Pepper
- Garlic powder

Method:

Step 1: Preheat the oven to 375 f. and Lightly Spray a flat pizza baking tray and sit to the side.

Step 2: In a large mixing bowl, add spelt flour, mixed herbs, a pinch of pink Himalayan salt.

Step 3: Then slowly add water and mix with a spoon, once dough starts to form, use your hands to kneed together.

Step 4: Form into a ball, place on a flat surface. Then use a rolling pin to roll dough into to a flat pizza like base.

Step 5: Using a fork pierce the flat bread all over, then place in the oven for 10-12 mins.

While your flat bread is in the oven. Start to prepare your Avocado.

Step 6: Peel and take out the seed from a large Avocado, place in a Medium size bowl.

Step 7: Add lime juice, Himalayan salt, black pepper, mixed herbs and mash with a fork, until guacamole texture.

Step 8: Once your flat bread is ready, remove from the oven, let cool for about 5 mins.

Step 9: Slice your bread in to squares or pizza shape slices, spread with avocado and Enjoy!

2. Fresh Fruit Salad

Ingredients:

- Organic Papaya
- Mango
- Organic Strawberries

Method:

Step 1: Wash and soak your strawberries in water and 2 capfuls of apple cider vinegar.

Step 2: Then peel your mango and papaya and cut into bite size pieces. Add to a medium size mixing bowl.

Step 3: If you have a shape cutter feel free to use it, to make things more fun for your little ones.

Step 4: Rinse your strawberries.

Step 5: Then and cut add to the bowl, mix up the chopped fruit and Enjoy!

3. Papaya Boat

Ingredients:

- 1 Papaya
- Agave
- 1 tbsp Almond Butter
- 1 Burro or Small banana
- 1 ½ tsp Hemp, chia, flax seeds
- ¼ tsp Cinnamon

Method:

Step 1: Rinse your papaya then cut into an equal half, wrap another half and store in the fridge if not going to use it.

Step 2: Scrape out many of the seeds (leaving a few) Store the remaining seeds in a container.

(The seeds are great to consume to clean out the gut and kill parasites).

Step 3: Then slice your banana and place in the center of the papaya.

Step 4: Then add hemp, chia, flax seeds.

Step 5: Then add Almond butter

Step 6: Sprinkle with cinnamon and drizzle with Agave.

Grab a spoon and Enjoy!

4. Açaí Bowl

Ingredients:

- Frozen Acai
- Frozen Mango
- ½ tbsp Agave
- 1 small Banana
- Fresh wild Blueberries
- Fresh Organic Strawberries
- Toppings of your choice (Shredded Coconut, hemp, flax, chia seeds, goji berries, almond butter)

Method:

Step 1: Wash and Soak Strawberries and Blueberries.

Step 2: Rinse well then slice Strawberries and Banana.

Step 3: Place Frozen Acai, frozen mango and agave in a high-speed Blender, blend into thick Ice-cream texture.

Step 4: Spoon into a bowl

Step 5: Nicely place the banana, strawberries and blueberries on top of the acai.

Step 6: Sprinkle on desired toppings, then drizzle with agave and Enjoy!

5. Breakfast Smoothie

Ingredients:

- 2 small Bananas
- ½ cup Frozen Blueberries
- Organic Kale
- 1 tsp Spirulina
- 125ml Fresh spring water
- 100ml Fresh Orange Juice
- 1 tsp Agave (optional)
- 2 tbp Kamut flakes (Optional)

Method:

Step 1: Place all of your ingredients in a high-speed blender.

Step 2: Blend until smoothie Juice texture.

Step 3: Pour into smoothie cups and Enjoy!

6. Maca Super Food Breakfast Muffins

Ingredients:

- 2 small Bananas
- 1 tbsp Maca Powder
- 1 tbsp Chia seed
- 1 Cup Spelt Flour
- 1/2 Cup Quinoa Flour
- 1/4 Cup buckwheat Flour
- 1 tsp Cinnamon
- 1 1/2 tsp Baking Powder
- 1/2 tsp Baking Soda
- 1/2 CUP Coconut Oil (melted)
- 1 Cup plant-based milk of your choice
- 5 tbsp Agave

Method:

Step 1: Mix all dry ingredients together in a bowl.

Step 2: Add All Liquids together in a blender, including the banana and blend.

Step 3: Add wet ingredients to the dry mixture and stir. Then set mixture aside.

Step 4: preheat oven to 375 degrees F

Step 5: Fill muffin cases equally using an Ice cream scooper if possible.

Step 6: Bake in the oven for 20-25mins or until toothpick inserted comes out clean.

7. Kamut porridge

Kamut is an Alkaline ancient grain that is much healthier than oats.

Ingredients:

- 1 ½ cup Kamut Grain
- 4 ½ cups Hemp Milk
- ¼ Cinnamon
- ¼ Nutmeg
- Agave
- 2 tbsp Sea moss Gel (optional)
- Pinch of Himalayan Salt
- 1 tsp Vanilla
- 2 cups spring water

Method:

- **Step 1:** Soak kamut overnight in about 2 cups of water.

- **Step 2:** Cook the kamut a little, about 10 minutes and let cool.

- **Step 3:** Blend kamut with the same water you used to cook it. If you want the consistency smooth, blend for longer.

- **Step 4:** Add hemp milk to blender.

- **Step 5:** Add all the other ingredients except agave and blend for a few seconds.

- **Step 6:** Cook mixture on medium heat for 20 minutes (stir continuously to avoid lumps).

- **Step 7:** Add agave and Enjoy!

Chapter 7

2 WEEKS OF KIDS PACKED LUNCH

WEEK 1:

MONDAY	TUESDAY	WEDNESDAY	THURSAY	FRIDAY
Lunch: Hummus with Chia Seed or grain crackers, with sliced Cucumbers and Fresh Strawberries.	**Lunch:** Avocado Dip, Spelt flat bread, Celery sticks and unsweet-ened blueberry applesauce.	**Lunch:** Chickpea "TUNA" sandwich on spelt bread, apple slices and Blueberries.	**Lunch:** Avocado Quinoa Salad, Grapes and apple sauce.	**Lunch:** Jamaican Spin-ach or vegetable Patty, Fresh Sliced Mango and Strawberries.
Snack: Applesauce and Lara bar or raw fruit Bar.	**Snack:** Diced Mango and sea salt Veggie Straw Chips.	**Snack:** Baby Banana and organic raisins.	**Snack:** Clif Kid organic Zbar.	**Snack:** Lightly salted Green Banana Chips.

Drink:	Drink:	Drink:	Drink:	Drink:
8 FLoz Bottled Spring Water and "Honest" Grape organic Juice Drink.	8 FLoz Spring water And "Honest" Apple organic Juice Drink.	8 FL oz Spring Water And "Honest" Fruit punch organic Juice Drink.	8 FL oz Spring water and " Honest" Berry Lemonade organic Juice Drink.	8 FL oz Spring Water and ' "Honest" Grape organic Juice Drink.
Tip:	**Tip:**	**Tip:**	Tip:	Tip:
Adjust accordingly, you may substitute, add or subtract as you please.	Spelt Flat bread is normally home-made. This can be substituted if needed.	Readymade spelt bread can be found at wholefoods.	With salad or anything that needs to be kept cold, place icepack in lunch bag.	Jamaican veg patty can be found any Caribbean restaurant.

WEEK 2:

MONDAY	TUESDAY	WEDNESDAY	THURSDAY	FRIDAY
Lunch: Falafel & Hummus wrap, Fresh Blueberries and Strawberries.	**Lunch:** Avocado Dip, Grain Cracker, Red Pepper, celery and Cucumber.	**Lunch:** small bowl of mixed diced fruit, Pineapple, mango and Strawberry. Sweet hummus-snickerdoodle, vegan pretzels.	**Lunch:** crispy Quinoa Bites, organic vegan ketchup, chickpea salad.	**Lunch:** Vegan Blueberry Muffin, Strawberry Coconut Milk Yogurt, Fresh Grapes.
Snack: Sea Salt Veggie Straw Chips.	**Snack:** Home-Made Superfood Muffin.	**Snack:** Clif kids organic fruit twist	**Snack:** Applesauce and Lara bar.	**Snack:** Terra Blues- Purple sweet potato chips.

Drink: 8 FL oz Bottled Spring water and "Honest" Organic Juice Drink.	Drink: 8 FL oz Spring water and "Honest" Berry Lemonade organic Juice Drink.	Drink: 8 FL oz Spring water And "Honest" Apple organic Juice Drink.	Drink: 8 FL oz Spring Water and "Honest" Grape organic Juice Drink.	Drink: 8 FL oz Spring Water And "Honest" Fruit punch organic Juice Drink.
Tip: Some of These Items listed are store bought, but can be home-made.	Tip: Avocado or Hummus single dips can be found at any grocery store.	Tip: Dessert Hummus can be found at grocery stores such as Publix.	Tip: Quinoa veggie bites can be homemade or store brought. Find in the fresh veggie isle.	Tip: Brands such as "So Delicious" and "silk" have dairy free yogurt options.

Note: Make Lunch time for your kids more fun by cutting fruit into special shapes, or by popping little Fun notes in their lunch boxes.

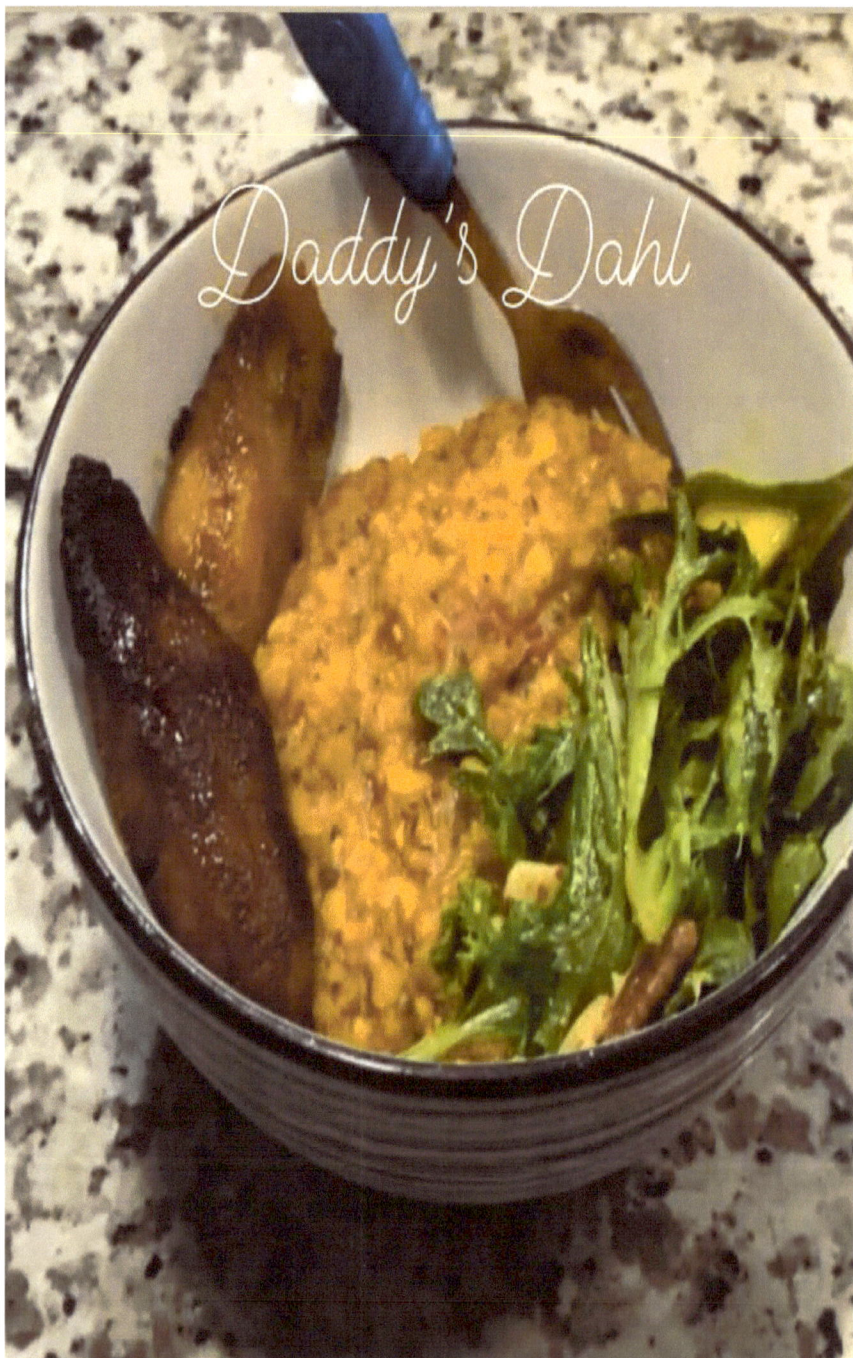

Daddy's Dahl

Chapter 8

14 DAYS OF PLANT-BASED DINNER RECIPES

Note: All recipes are listed to serve roughly around a family of 4. You can adjust measurements to your preference.

Most of these Recipes use **Alkaline** vegan ingredients.

Try stay away from canned products. Soak chickpeas over night or you can purchase them already cooked in a box package or even a pouch. Always rinse before using.

Always Clean your fruit and vegetables before use. I use apple cider to clean my fruits and vegetables.

DAY 1 - VEGAN PASTA WITH BUTTERNUT SQUASH SAUCE.

Ingredients:

1 bag of precut butternut squash 340g bag.

1 small onion

4 garlic cloves

1 Tube or carton of organic Tomato purée

1 zucchini

Spinach

1/2 Red bell Pepper

Sea Salt

Black pepper

Mixed herbs

Basil

Spelt Penne Pasta or Quinoa Spaghetti (or pasta of choice)

Method:

Step 1: Boil butternut squash for 15-20 mins until fork tender.

Step 2: Meanwhile, chop all veggies including spinach.

Step 3: Boil a Large pot of water for the pasta.

Step 4: In a large pan add a little grape seed oil or a little spring water and sauté on medium heat, add half of the chopped garlic, half of the chopped onion and ALL the chopped zucchini and spinach. Until tender.

For The Sauce:

Step1: Add to your blender, Tomato purée, all the remaining chopped veggies, 3/4 of cooked butternut squash (save the rest of the cooked precut squash to add in the pan), add sea salt, black pepper, mixed herbs, fresh basil.

Step 2: Then add 115ml of spring water, Blend together.

If needed, add more water or squash to reach your desired sauce texture.

Step 5: Then add sauce to the sautéed veggies in the pot. Stir well.

Step 6: Add in the remaining cooked butter-nut squash.

Step 7: (Cook pasta according to the package instructions) Then add cooked pasta to the pot and stir. Let Simmer for 2-3 mins and Enjoy!

Tips: Taste sauce and add additional seasoning if necessary.

DAY 2- QUINOA STIR FRY

Ingredients:

1 cup pre-cooked cooled quinoa

1 tablespoon grapeseed oil

1 teaspoon sesame seed oil

1/2 cup minced green onions

2 cloves garlic, minced

1/2 Bell pepper red/green

1-2 stalks of Bok Choy

1-2 stalks of Kale

5-6 diced Mushrooms

5 tablespoons Bragg Liquid coconut Amino, to taste

Pink Himalayan Salt optional

1/2 tsp Onion powder

1 tsp Chinese 5 spice

2tbp Agave

Instructions:

Step 1: Pre heat wok with oil Add 3/4 green onions, peppers to the pan and sauté over a medium heat for a few minutes until just starting to soften.

Step 2: Then add the mushrooms chopped kale and bok choy Cook for another couple of minutes.

Step 3: While cooking mix in the liquid amino with the agave, salt and Chinese 5 spice in a small bowl

Step 4: Add the cooked quinoa to the pan along with the sauce mixture.

Step 5: Stir together well and cook until the quinoa is heated through.

Step 6: Serve sprinkled with the remaining green onions and Enjoy!

DAY 3- COCONUT CHICKPEA CURRY

Ingredients:

1 tbsp grapeseed oil

1 large red onion thinly sliced

3 cloves garlic minced

1-inch fresh ginger peeled and minced

1 tbsp garam masala

2 tbsp Curry powder

1/4 tsp cayenne pepper (or to taste)

1/4 tsp pink Himalayan salt (plus more to taste)

1 and 1/2 cups diced tomatoes

1 and 1/2 cups full-fat coconut milk

1 and 3/4 cups cooked chickpeas

2 tbsp freshly-squeezed lime juice

chopped fresh cilantro (coriander)

Instructions:

Step 1: In a large pan, heat the grapeseed oil over medium-high heat. Add the red onion with a pinch of salt. Cook, stirring frequently, until the onion is softened and starting to brown.

Step 2: Reduce the heat to medium. Add the garlic and ginger; stir and cook for a minute. Stir in the garam masala, curry powder, and salt. Cook for 30 seconds more to toast the spices.

Step 3: Add the tomatoes to the pan and stir well. Continue to cook, stirring occasionally, for about 3-5 minutes or until the tomatoes are starting to break down and dry up a little bit. Stir in the coconut milk and chickpeas. Bring the mixture to a boil, then reduce the heat to medium-low.

Step 4: Simmer the coconut chickpea curry for about 10 minutes or until reduced slightly. Stir in the fresh lime juice. Season to taste with additional salt (I used about another 1/2 teaspoon at this point). Serve hot, over quinoa or wild rice or grain of choice, and garnished with chopped fresh cilantro.

DAY 4- VEGGIE BURGER PATTY'S WITH HOMEMADE FRIES.

Ingredients:

1 cup Garbanzo Bean Flour

1/2 cup Onions, diced

1/2 cup Green Peppers, diced

1/2 cup Kale, diced

1 Plum Tomato, diced

2 tsp. Basil

2 tsp. Oregano

2 tsp. Onion Powder

2 tsp. Sea Salt

1 tsp. Dill

1/2 tsp. Ginger Powder

1/2 tsp. Cayenne Powder

1/4 to 1/2 cup Spring Water

Grape Seed Oil

Sweet potato or regular potato

Avocado mayo

1/2 lime

Instructions:

Step 1: Preheat oven to 375 f

Step 2: Peel and cut potato into fries

Step 3: Place in a baking tray, drizzle some grapeseed oil and sprinkle with a pinch of salt and oregano.

Bake for 30mins or until golden.

Step 4: In a large bowl, mix together all seasonings and vegetables, then mix in flour.

Slowly add water and mix until mixture can be formed into a patty. Add more flour if too loose.

Step 5: Add oil to skillet and cook patties on medium-high heat for 2-3 minutes on each side. Continue flipping until both sides are brown.

Step 6: Peel and mash avocado, add lime, salt, onion powder, grapeseed oil, oregano. Mix into mayo texture.

DAY 5: VEGAN PIZZA

There are some great vegan pizza options at Whole Foods. Either you can get it made fresh or buy the frozen option for when you have those busy rushed days.

Here's a recipe for those who would like to make a pizza from scratch:

Ingredients:

1 ½ Spelt flour

1 cup Spring water

Puréed plum tomatoes

½ tsp Basil

½ tsp oregano

½ tsp Sea salt

1 tsp Key lime

Toppings:

Mushrooms

Kale

Cheese- daiya shredded (optional) or Walnut cheese.

(Soaked walnuts (2 hours in hot water), onion powder, sea salt, pepper flakes, lime)

Instructions:

Step 1: For the crust: mix ingredients and press out the crust to your desired thickness. Use a fork to poke holes in the crust.

Step 2: For the sauce: place ingredients in blender. Cook on medium heat until sauce thickens or reaches desired consistency.

Step 3: For the Walnut cheese: put all ingredients in a food processor and pulse a few times.

Or use vegan cheeses such as daiya shredded.

Step 4: Bake the crust for 8-10 minutes, add sauce and toppings and bake another 10-12mintues with the last few minutes under the broiler.

Enjoy!

DAY 6- BAKED POTATO WITH CHICKPEA SALAD.

Ingredients:

4 Regular potato or sweet potato

½ tsp Vegan butter

175 cups Cooked Chickpeas

1 Spring onion

1/4 Cucumber

1/4 tsp Onion powder

1 tsp Olive oil or coconut oil

1/4 tsp Oregano

1/4 tsp Pink Himalayan salt

1/4 lime

Instructions:

Step 1: Preheat oven to 375 f

Step 2: Wash potato and pierce with a fork. Rub with some grape seed oil and bake for 30-35 mins.

Step 3: Finely Chop spring onion, Red onion and cucumber.

Step 4: Place cooked chickpeas into a mixing bowl add onions, Spring onion and cucumber.

Step 5: Then add dry seasoning and oil and mix.

Step 6: Once potato is ready, poke with fork to ensure inside is soft.

Step 7: Using a sharp knife cut potato in the middle. Using a fork scrape the sides add butter and a pinch of salt and oregano and lightly mash together.

Step 8: Then serve along with the chickpea salad and Enjoy!

DAY7- VEGAN PESTO PASTA

Ingredients:

Pesto:

1 1/2 cups packed basil

1/2 cup packed flat leaf Italian parsley

1 cup green peas (if frozen, thawed)

4 cloves garlic (4 cloves yield ~2 Tbsp)

1/4 cup toasted pine nuts (plus more for serving // or sub raw walnuts, but omit as garnish)

1 lime, juiced (~2 Tbsp or 30 ml per lime)

1/4 cup vegan parmesan cheese (plus more for serving)

1 pinch sea salt (plus more to taste)

1/4 cup olive oil

Pasta

10 ounces spelt penne pasta

1 Tbsp olive oil

2 cloves garlic, chopped

1/4 cup sun-dried tomatoes, chopped

1 cup chopped kale (optional)

Pink Himalayan Salt

Instructions:

Step1: Fill a large saucepan 3/4 full of water, salt generously, and bring to a boil.

Step2: In the meantime, prepare pesto. To a food processor, add basil, parsley, peas, garlic, pine nuts, lime juice, vegan parmesan cheese and sea salt. Mix to combine. While the machine is running, stream in olive oil through the spout.

Step 3: Continue blending, scraping down sides as needed, until creamy and fully combined. If it has trouble blending add a bit more olive oil or water.

Step 4: Taste and adjust seasonings as needed, add more lime juice if necessary, vegan parmesan for cheesy flavor.

Step5: Next add pasta to boiling water and cook according to package instructions. Be sure not to overcook and drain when pasta still have a slight bite to them. Take off heat and set aside.

Step 6: Once your pasta is drained, heat a large saucepan over medium heat. Once hot, add grapeseed oil, garlic, and sun-dried tomatoes and kale. Sauté for 1-2 minutes, or until the garlic is fragrant but not yet browned.

Step 7: Turn off heat and remove skillet from stove, then add cooked pasta and toss to coat.

Step 8: Transfer to a serving platter or mixing bowl and add 3/4 of the pesto. Toss to combine.

Step 9: Serve warm with additional pesto on the side, and garnish generously with additional parsley, pine nuts, and vegan parmesan cheese.

Best when fresh, though leftovers will keep in the refrigerator up to 2-3 days. Enjoy!

DAY 8- CARIBBEAN SPLIT PEA SOUP

Ingredients:

1 small onion

4 cloves garlic

1 celery stalk

2 small red potatoes

1 large carrot (optional)

1 green banana

2/3 cup split peas [tip: I used dried Goya peas and did not soak overnight. no worries just add the peas to 3-4 cups of hot water and boil for 2 minutes. let stand for 1 hour then drain and rinse. the peas will be slightly softened, and will continue to soften as you cook the soup]

2 leaves kale

4 cups vegetable stock + 2 cups water

1 Tsp avocado oil

Spices: Thyme, allspice, cumin, bonnet pepper (optional), cayenne pepper, pink Himalayan salt

Dumplings

1 1/2 cup spelt flour

1 Tbs cold butter

1/2 cup cold water

Instructions:

Step 1: In a large pot, add olive oil over medium heat

Step 2: Once oil is heated, add chopped onion, celery, and garlic. Stir until softened [about 5 minutes]

Step 3: Stir in allspice, thyme, black pepper, pepper powder, and cumin, stirring consistently for 1 minute. Leave the seasoning salt for the end so you can season to taste.

Step 4: Peel and chop vegetables. Add vegetables & chopped plantain to pot and stir until all ingredients are combined.

Step 5: Add vegetable stock and water to pot.

Step 6: Add split peas.

Step 7: Remove kale leaves from the steam rinse and chop into small pieces, then add to the soup

Bring soup to a boil, then reduce the heat to medium-low for 35 mins.

Now for the dumplings:

Step 1: Place the flour in a bowl.

Step 2: Using your fingers, break the butter into small pieces and crumble into flour mixture.

Step 3: Pour water into bowl, a little at a time! Begin combining the flour and water until it reaches slightly sticky consistency. You don't want to over work the flour mixture.

Step 4: Pinch a piece of dough and Roll the dough between the palm of the hands into dumpling shape.

When there is 20 minutes left, drop the dumplings into the soup and left finish cooking. Stir occasionally so that the dumplings do not stick to the bottom of the pot and Enjoy!

DAY 9- FALAFEL AND HUMMUS.

Ingredients:

To make 30 balls:

1 lb. dry chickpeas/garbanzo beans - you must start with dry, do NOT substitute canned, they will not work!

1 small onion, roughly chopped

1/4 cup chopped fresh parsley

3-5 cloves garlic (I prefer roasted garlic cloves)

1 1/2 tbsp flour or chickpea flour

1 3/4 tsp salt

2 tsp cumin

1 tsp ground coriander

1/4 tsp black pepper

1/4 tsp cayenne pepper

Pinch of ground cardamom

Grapeseed oil for frying

1 cup cooked Quinoa

1 Avocado

½ Cucumber

1 tub of premade Organic Hummus

Instructions:

Step 1: Pour the chickpeas into a large bowl and cover them by about 3 inches of cold water. Let them soak overnight. They will double in size as they soak – you will have between 4 and 5 cups of beans after soaking.

Step 2: Drain and rinse the garbanzo beans well. Pour them into your food processor along with the chopped onion, garlic cloves, parsley, flour or chickpea flour (use chickpea flour to make gluten free), salt, cumin, ground coriander, black pepper, cayenne pepper, and cardamom. NOTE: if you have a smaller food processor, you will want to divide the ingredients in half and process the mixture one batch at a time.

Step 3: Pulse all ingredients together until a rough, coarse meal forms. Scrape the sides of the processor periodically and push the mixture down the sides. Process till the mixture is somewhere between the texture of couscous and a paste. You want the mixture to hold together, and a more paste-like consistency will help with that... but don't over process, you don't want it turning into hummus!

Step 4: Once the mixture reaches the desired consistency, pour it out into a bowl and use a fork to stir; this will make the texture more even throughout. Remove any large chickpea chunks that the processor missed.

Step 5: Cover the bowl with plastic wrap and refrigerate for 1-2 hours.

Note: Some people like to add baking soda to the mix to lighten up the texture inside of the falafel balls. I don't usually add it, since the falafel is generally fluffy on its own. If you would like to add it, dissolve 2 tsp of baking soda in 1 tbsp of water and mix it into the falafel mixture after it has been refrigerated.

Step 6: Fill a skillet with grapeseed oil to a depth of 1 ½ inches. Heat the oil slowly over medium heat. The ideal temperature to fry falafel is between 360- and 375-degrees F; the best way to monitor the temperature is to use a deep fry or candy thermometer. After making these a few times, you will start to get a feel for when the oil temperature is "right."

Step 7: Meanwhile, form falafel mixture into round balls or slider-shaped patties using wet hands or a falafel scoop.

I usually use about 2 tbsp of mixture per falafel. You can make them smaller or larger depending on your personal preference. The balls will stick together loosely at first but will bind nicely once they begin to fry.

Note: If the balls won't hold together, place the mixture back in the processor again and continue processing to make it more paste-like. Keep in mind that the balls will be delicate at first; if you can get them into the hot oil, they will bind together and stick. If they still won't hold together, you can try adding 2-3 tbsp chickpea flour to the mixture.

Step 8: When the oil is at the right temperature, fry the falafels in batches of 5-6 at a time till golden brown on both sides. 2-3 minutes each side.

Step 9: Once the falafels are fried, remove them from the oil using a slotted spoon.

Step 10: Place on paper towels. Serve the falafels fresh and hot with hummus and I normally do a quinoa Avocado salad. You can also stuff them into a pita.

Quinoa Avocado salad

Step 1: Dice cucumber and avocado into small cube like pieces.

Step 2: place cooked quinoa, cucumber, avocado, seasoning, lime and oil of choice in a mixing bowl.

Step 3: Mix together and Enjoy!

DAY 10 - VEGAN LASAGNA

Ingredients:

Spelt Lasagna Sheets

Tomato Sauce:

12 Plum Tomatoes

1 tbsp. Agave

1 tbsp. Onion Powder

2 tsp. Basil

2 tsp. Oregano

2 tsp. Sea Salt

1/2 tsp. Cayenne Powder

1 cup Onions, Chopped

1 cup Green, Yellow, and Red Peppers, diced

2 tbsp. Onion Powder

1 tbsp. Sea Salt

2 tsp. Oregano

2 tsp. Basil

Zucchini

1 stalk kale

5 White Mushrooms

9x13 Glass Baking Dish

Grape Seed Oil

Brazil Nut Cheese:

2 cups Soaked Brazil Nuts

1 cup Spring Water

1 tbsp. Hemp Seeds

1 tbsp. Onion Powder

1 tsp. Sea Salt

1 tsp. Oregano

1 tsp. Basil

½ Lime

Instructions:

Step 1: Blend together all tomato sauce ingredients in a blender until well blended.

Step 2: Add to a saucepan at medium heat and bring to a boil, then simmer sauce on a low heat, stirring occasionally, for 45 mins or until it has thickened.

Step 3: Thinly slice mushrooms, kale and zucchini into small pieces

Step 4: On high heat, lightly oil skillet with grape seed oil and sauté onions and peppers for 5 minutes.

Step 5: Then add the mushrooms, kale and zucchini to the pan, sauté for another 3-4 minutes.

Step 6: Add 1 cup of spring water and all other cheese ingredients to blender and blend until mixed well. If too thick, add 1/4 cup more water at a time until desired consistency is reached.

Step 7: Begin building lasagna in glass dish by lightly coating bottom of the dish with tomato sauce. This is so the pasta doesn't stick to the pan.

Step 8: Lay in pasta, sautéed vegetable mix, cheese, then pasta once again. Repeat this step until you have 4 layers of pasta.

Step 9: Top off last layer of pasta with sautéed vegetables mix and cheese, then pour remaining tomato sauce around the lasagna. Optional: Lightly sprinkle with vegan shredded cheese and basil.

Step 10: Bake at 350°F for 35-45 minutes.

Allow to cool for 15 minutes before serving and enjoy!

DAY 11- VEGAN TACO BOWL

Ingredients:

1 cup quinoa

15 ounces cooked chickpeas

1 Tsp coconut oil

1 Tbsp Grape seed oil

Pink Himalayan salt

Oregano

Onion powder

Cilantro

GUACAMOLE

1 avocado ripe

1/2 lime juiced

Salt to taste

Cumin to taste

TOPPINGS

Plum tomato diced

Cilantro minced

Salsa

Mixed leafy greens

Hummus (optional)

Instructions:

Step 1: Rinse quinoa well in fine mesh strainer until water runs clear. Bring 2 cups of water to a rolling boil. Add quinoa and let simmer in lightly seasoned water for 15-20 minutes.

Step 2: Heat grapeseed oil in skillet over medium-high heat. Add chickpeas and season with seasoning. Heat 5-10 minutes, until warmed through.

Step 3: Place cooked quinoa in bowl and top with chickpeas. Assemble bowls as you like with desired toppings.

GUACAMOLE

Step 1: Mash avocado and lime juice with a fork. Season with a pinch of onion powder salt and cumin. Season to desired taste and Enjoy!

DAY 12- VEGAN LETTUCE WRAPS

Ingredients:

1 Avocado

1 cup walnuts

1 tbsp olive oil

1/2 onion, diced

1/2 Green pepper

1 clove of garlic

2 tbsp grapeseed or Avocado oil

1/4 cup liquid amino

½ Himalayan salt

½ tsp Onion powder

½ Oregano

Pinch Cayenne pepper (optional

Salsa

Instructions:

Step 1: In a food processor, pulse walnuts until you get a meat like texture. Set aside.

Step 2: Add grapeseed oil to pan over medium high heat. Once hot, sauté onions, green peppers and garlic for a few minutes, until soft.

Step 3: Add walnuts, amino and powder seasonings, mix until fully combined.

Step 4: rinse Romain leaf's, then Fill with walnut meat mixture and top with sliced avocado or guacamole and salsa. Enjoy!

DAY 13- DADDY'S VEGAN DAHL

Ingredients:

350g Red Lentils

900ml Vegetable stock

1 onion, chopped

2 cloves of garlic, minced

½ Lime

250g chopped plum Tomatoes

1tsp Turmeric

1 tsp cumin

½ tsp cayenne pepper

1 tsp coriander

1 tsp masala

½ cinnamon

1 tap pink Himalayan salt

Grain of choice rice or Quinoa

Method:

Step 1: Chop onion and garlic finely or blend in food processor.

Step 2: Fry onion and garlic until transparent, do not burn garlic.

Step 3: Add in plum Tomatoes and spices with a little water. Sautee

Step 4: Finally add in the rinsed lentils, stock and lime juice.

Step 5: Bring to a broil, then simmer for 20-22 minutes.

Step 6: Cook rice or quinoa according to package instructions, serve and Enjoy!

DAY 14- MUSHROOM POT ROAST WITH HERB ROAST POTATOES.

Ingredients:

4-5 Potatoes

4 large portobello mushrooms, sliced into pieces

1 large onion, sliced

2 cloves garlic, pressed

3 tablespoons spelt flour

1 teaspoon sage

1 teaspoon dried basil

3 cups vegetable broth, divided

4 potatoes, quartered

4 carrots, cut into 3-inch pieces

Salt and pepper, to taste

2 teaspoons liquid amino

3 sprigs fresh thyme

1 sprig fresh rosemary

Pastry (optional)

1 1/2 Spelt flour

1/2 cup Vegan butter or coconut oil

7-9 tbsp of cold Water

1/2 tsp coconut sugar

1/2 tsp salt

Instructions:

Step 1: Preheat oven to 375degrees.

Step 2: Peel and cut potatoes into desired size.

Step 3: Boil for 10-15mins, then strain.

Step 4: Place in a baking tray drizzle with oil pinch of salt and mixed herbs.

Then Set a side.

Step 6: In a large saucepan, heat grape-seed oil and add portobello mushroom slices. Allow to cook through and brown a bit—you'll need to keep moving them around and turning them—and then remove from pan and set aside.

Step 7: Then add onion and garlic. Caramelize onions by stirring until they wilt and begin to brown. Remove onions from pan and set aside.

Step 8: Mix spelt flour, sage, and basil together in a small bowl. Stir in ¼ cup of broth to create a paste and pour mixture into the same pan you used for mushrooms and onions. While stirring constantly over medium heat, slowly add remaining broth to create a sauce.

Step 9: When mixture starts to boil, turn off heat and add any additional seasonings. Add potatoes, carrots, salt, pepper, and Liquid amino to the sauce. If more liquid is needed to keep the vegetables from drying out, add more broth.

Step 10: Add mushrooms and onions to mixture and ladle into a large ceramic or glass deep pie or casserole dish, layering rosemary and thyme. Add lid, place pan into oven, and bake for 50 mins

If using pastry crust on top:

Step 1: Combine flours, sugar, and salt in a large bowl and whisk together. Add solid coconut oil to bowl and using your fingertips rub the coconut oil into the dry ingredients until the mixture begins to form fine crumbs (it will look like wet sand).

Step 2: Add ice water to flour mixture 1 tablespoon at a time and use a wooden spoon to gently mix. Continue to add water (no more than 9 tablespoons) and mix until a dough form.

Step 3: Using a rolling pin, roll out large enough to cover the top of the baking dish, allow excess edges to hang.

Fold the excess edges back over to form the crust.

Step 4: Pierce the center of the pot pie with a fork.

Step 5: Place in the oven. Bake for 45-50mins or until crust is golden.

Step 6: The remaining 30 mins, place the potatoes on the second shelf and bake until golden crisp.

Remove from oven and serve Pot Roast with herb roast potatoes and veg of your choice. Enjoy!

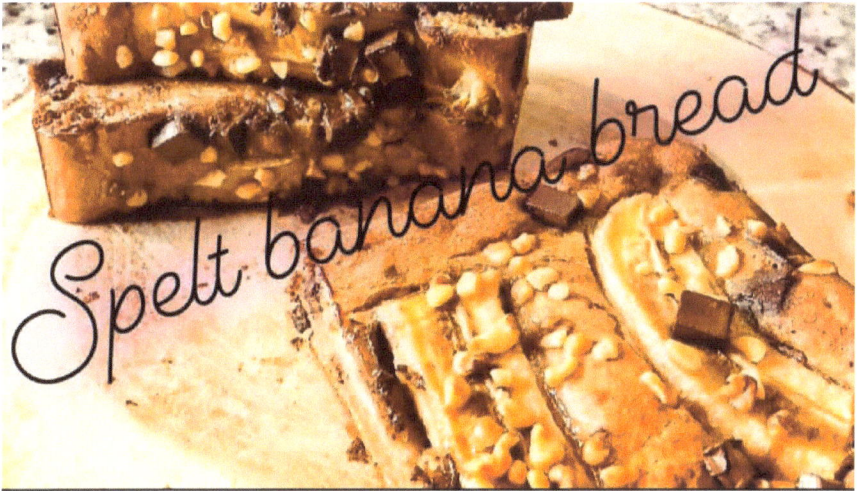

Spelt banana bread

Chapter 9

PLANT-BASED DESSERTS

Some people may think that being vegan, means you must miss out on delicious desserts. I can assure you that you can still enjoy your old favorites, without any guilt.

I am going to provide you with my Top five Vegan dessert recipes, that my family and I enjoy.

1. Vegan Banana Nice-Cream

Ingredients:

6-7 Frozen Baby Bananas

1 cup of frozen mango or fruit of your choice(optional)

½ cup Coconut Milk

2-3 tsp of Spirulina (adds fun color optional)

Method:

Step 1: Place all ingredients in a Food Processor or high- speed blender.

Step 2: Blend until thick ice cream texture appears.

Don't over blend or Ice cream texture will become to runny.

Step 3: Scoop into a bowl, Top with fresh of your Choice and Enjoy!

2. **Key Lime Tart**

Ingredients:

Crust-

- 12 Vegan Graham crackers
- 5 tbsp Coconut oil
- 9 Dates (pitted)
- Key Lime Zest (from 2 key limes)
- 1 ½ tsp Pink Himalayan salt

Filling-

- 3 Avocados
- 1 cup raw Cashew (Soaked Overnight)

- 1 tsp Coconut oil
- ¼ cup triple filtered coconut oil
- 1¾ cup Lime Juice
- 1 cup Agave
- 1 tbsp Vanilla extract

Method:

Step 1: Place graham crackers in the food processor and blend, then add coconut oil, dates, key lime zest and pink Himalayan salt, blend into a fine sand-like texture.

Step 2: Press mixture into a 9inch spring form pan, press evenly and set in the freezer until filling mixture is ready.

Step 3: Then add Avocados, soaked cashews, coconut oil, key Lime Juice, vanilla extract and agave, process until thick creamy smooth texture.

Step 4: Add filling to the crust, smooth out evenly with an icing spatula.

Step 5: Place in freezer for 3-4 hours

Step 6: Top with Coconut whipped cream (Optional) and Enjoy!

3. **Cherry Bakewell Chia Seed Pudding**

Ingredients:

- ¼ cup of Chia Seeds
- 1 cup Coconut or hemp Milk (or Plant based milk of your choice)
- ½ tsp Almond extract
- Dark Sweet pitted Cherries (frozen or fresh)
- 2 burro or small Bananas
- 1 tbsp Agave

Method:

Step 1: First chop bananas, then place at the bottom of dessert glasses or cups.

Step 2: Then add frozen cherries or fresh cherries, set to the side.

Step 3: Place chia seeds in a mixing bowl, add plant-based milk, almond extract and agave.

Step 4: Mix well, then pour chia seed pudding mixture on top of the already prepared cherries and bananas.

Step 5: Set in fridge for 1-2 hours or overnight for best results, Then Enjoy!

4. Spelt Banana Bread.

Ingredients:

- 5-6 ripe burro or small bananas
- 1 ½ cups Spelt Flour
- 1/3 cup Hemp milk
- 3 tbsp Agave
- ¼ cup Date sugar
- ½ tsp Cinnamon
- ½ Nutmeg
- 2 tbsp Ground flaxseed
- 1/3 cup coconut oil (melted)
- 2 tsp vanilla extract
- 1 tsp baking soda
- ½ tsp baking powder
- ½ tsp Pink Himalayan salt
- Chopped Walnuts (Optional)

Method:

Step1: Preheat Oven to 350 f. Lightly grease a 9x5 loaf baking pan.

Set to the side and start to prepare mixture.

Step 2: In a large mixing bowl mash the bananas until a smooth texture.

Step 3: Then add the melted coconut oil, hemp milk, ground flax, agave and vanilla extract. Mix well, then add in the dry ingredients date sugar, salt, baking powder, baking soda and spelt flour. Mix well.

Step4: Then spoon the batter into the loaf pan and smooth out evenly.

Step 5: Sprinkle walnuts on top a gentle press into the batter.

Step 6: Place in oven and bake for 45-55 minutes (Time may vary so keep an eye out) until firm on top and it's a light golden color.

Step 7: Take out of the oven and place on a cooling rack for 30 minutes.

Step 8: Using a knife gently take banana bread out of the pan and place directly on the cooling rack, until completely cooled.

Slice and Enjoy!

5. Vegan Donuts

Ingredients:

- 1/2 Almond Flour
- 1 cup Spelt Flour
- 1 tsp Tapioca Flour
- 2 tbsp Date Sugar
- ¼ tsp nutmeg
- Pink Himalayan salt (Pinch)
- 1 tsp Baking Powder
- 1 tsp Baking Soda
- 1 tsp Vanilla Extract
- 10 pitted Dates
- ½ cup Coconut milk
- 1/3 cup unsweetened apple sauce
- 1 tbsp apple cider vinegar
- Vegan Chocolate of your choice

Method:

Step 1: Preheat your oven to 350 f and prepare your donut shaped baking tray. Lightly spray to prevent sticking.

Step 2: Place all the dry Ingredients in the food processor and blend.

Step 3: Then add dates and blend again, then add all your wet ingredients, blend until you get a smooth batter.

Step 4: Spoon your batter into the baking tray, make sure you distribute evenly.

Step 5: Place in the oven and bake for 20-25 mins or until toothpick inserted comes out clean.

Step 6: Remove from oven and gently turn baking tray onto cooling rack.

Leave to cool before glazing with melted Vegan chocolate.

Step 7: Melt Vegan chocolate of your choice, once completely melted dip one side of the donut into chocolate. Then place back on the cooling rack to set. Let set for about 20 minutes until chocolate is hardened and Enjoy!

Chapter 10

KIDS YOGA

Practicing Yoga with your little ones is such a rewarding gesture. You could either enroll them in professional yoga classes or teach them yourself. It's an amazing idea to add Yoga in their routine, because there is so many proven benefits from simple Yoga exercises.

Studies show that yoga practice reduces problem behavior, reduces anxiety, increases focus, improve academic performance, improves posture, builds self-confidence and helps with emotional balance.

I Highly recommend you trying out some simple yoga poses with your kids; you can even do it from the comfort of your own home.

Find a quite area, get a yoga mat, and start with some of these simple poses below.

1. **"Snake" Kid's Yoga Pose**- Great for Opening back and Strengthens Chest.

2. **"Dog" Kid's Yoga Pose-** Strengthens arms and Legs, stretches arms, calves and hamstrings.

3. **"Happy Baby" Kid's Yoga Pose**- relives tension in lower back, stretches spine, calms the brain.

4. **"Airplane" Kid's Yoga Pose**- This is a great balancing pose, helps develop concentration, improves balance, builds core strength.

5. **"Eagle" Kid's Yoga Pose**- stretches upper back and shoulders, strengthens legs, ankles and hips, increases balance.

6. **"Child's pose" Kid's Yoga Pose**- Reduces stress and fatigue, relieves back, shoulder, neck and hip strain, helps circulation to the muscles and the joints of the back.

7. **"Triangle" Kid's Yoga pose**- Improves digestion and constipation, stimulates abdominal organ function, relieves stress, strengthens legs, knees, abdominals and back.

8. **"Swan" Kid's Yoga Pose**- Heart opening pose, increases flexibility, strengthens spine, shoulders

and arms, elevates mood, stretches shoulder, belly, and chest muscles.

9. **"Easy pose" Kid's Yoga Pose-** reduces anxiety, strengthens back, stretches knees and ankles.

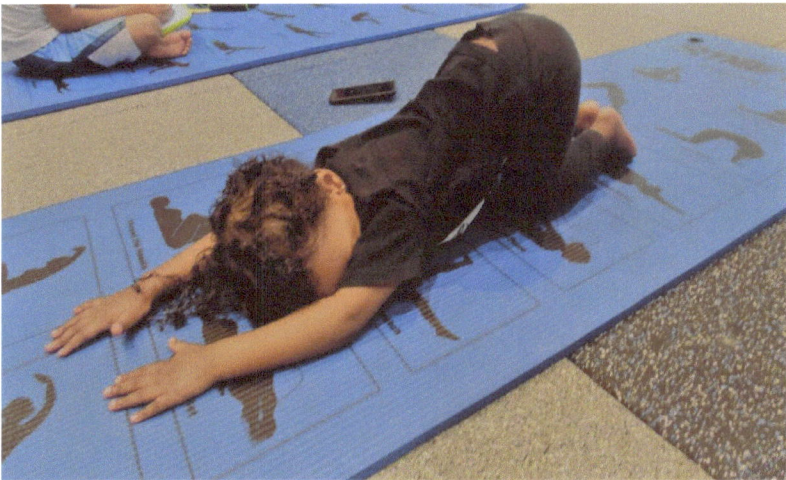

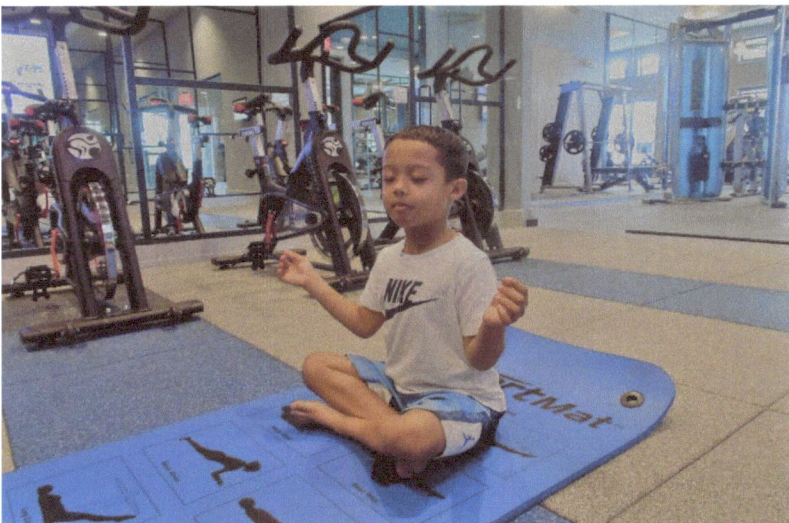

Chapter 11

MEDITATION AND PRAYER

As time goes on it seems easier and easier to be detached from spirituality. Teaching your kids from young, how to keep in balance and in control by simply take a few moments to meditate. This helps them to set positive intentions for the day, no matter the circumstance. Meditating has many other great benefits, and proven studies have shown that meditation; reduces tensions, helps with focus, helps with creative, social and alethic performance, mindfulness, access to natural rhythm of self-aware-ness, helps with overcoming negative emotions, increases compassion, improves child's attention span, and builds self-Love.

I believe both Prayer and Meditation are both important, there is a difference between the two. My personal explanation would be, Prayer is a way to connect and seek God. Mediation is a way to connect and find inner peace, which allows God to connect to you.

Simply find a quiet area and have your child or children get into the "Butterfly position". You can incorporate some mediation back ground music or use guided meditation. I will share a few of my favorites to use which come in handy, especially with the younger ages.

Remember practice makes perfect, and practice takes time. Your little ones might take a little time to get into it and get completely focus, but consistency is the key.

Teaching your kids to get into the habit of pray before bed, is a great way to wind down from the day and be Thankful for all blessings in life.

You can go on YouTube to find my top three background music suggestions for meditating. In the search bar type in "Deep Sea", "Charka Healing" and "Deep Mediation for kids". If you would like to use guided meditation, I will share some free links that I found helpful for the kid meditation.

Snowman Relaxation: hhtp://www.adoreyoga.com/_literature_104676/snowman_Relaxation_for_kids.mp3

Children's Rainbow Meditation- https://m.down-loadatoz.com/5-mintue-meditation/uk.co.olsonapps.fivemintuemeditation/

Mindful breathing- https://samharris.org/guided -meditations-for-children/

Guided Relaxation- http://www.fragrantheart.com/cms/free-audio-meditations/relaxation/relaxation -for-children

Magic Book Relaxation- https://www.excelatlife.com/mp3/magicbookmusic.mp3

Bouncing Ball Mindfulness- https://www.excelatlife.com/mp3/ball.mp3

Magic Forest- https://www.excelatlife.com/mp3/for-estmusic.mp3

Whirly Snowman storm meditation- https://www.cosmickids.com/mindfulness-meditation-videos-kids/

I Pray that this book was able to guide you through nutrition, exercise and useful tips of developing a positive mind set. I hope that it inspired you and your family to take a happier and healthier conscious eating path. May God Continue to guide you on your Journey to truth.

Thank you for your support.

Peace and Love
Joanna Walker